The Es... Air Fryer Cookbook

GW00499869

Recipes for Frying, Baking, Roasting, and Cooking Your Family's Favorite Meals

By

Elena Brown

This document is geared towards providing exact and reliable information in regards to the topic and issue covered. The publication is sold with the idea that the publisher is not required to render accounting, officially permitted or otherwise qualified services. If advice is necessary, legal or professional, a practiced individual in the profession should be ordered.

From a Declaration of Principles which was accepted and approved equally by a Committee of the American Bar Association and a Committee of Publishers and Associations.

In no way is it legal to reproduce, duplicate, or transmit any part of this document in either electronic means or in printed format. Recording of this publication is strictly prohibited, and any storage of this document is not allowed unless with written permission from the publisher. All rights reserved.

The information provided herein is stated to be truthful and consistent, in that any liability, in terms of inattention or otherwise, by any usage or abuse of any policies, processes, or directions contained within is the solitary and utter responsibility of the recipient reader. Under no circumstances will any legal responsibility or blame be held against the publisher for any reparation, damages, or *monetary loss due to the information herein, either directly or indirectly.*

Respective authors own all copyrights not held by the publisher.

The information herein is offered for informational purposes solely and is universal as so. The presentation of the information is without a contract or any type of guarantee assurance.

The trademarks used are without any consent, and the publication of the trademark is without permission or backing by the trademark owner. All trademarks and brands within this book are for clarifying purposes only and are owned by the owners themselves, not affiliated with this document.

Table of Contents

Introduction

The main advantage of air fryers is the possibility that people who thought they would never be able to enjoy French fries or croquettes from a fryer again may be able to eat them and have their sensitive stomachs tolerate them. Cooking without oil is healthier and possible with the best air fryers.

Easy to use. As a general rule, the operating panels of air fryers are clear and easy to use, highlighting the multiple functions and powers to best suit our tastes.

No fumes or odors. Air fryers emit fewer fumes and odors when cooking. This point is important when buying this type of appliance: the smell of fried food is quite difficult to get out of clothes and quite unpleasant when entering the house.

Cleanliness. The parts of air fryers, contrary to what it might seem because of their revolutionary cooking system, are easy to clean. Most of these machines are made up of parts that are easy to wash and can even be put in the dishwasher.

Savings. With just one tablespoon of oil, you can cook up to 1 kilo of potatoes. Oil is a basic element in Mediterranean and world cuisine. However, with an air fryer, it is possible to save the money that oil bottles cost. Think about it, a 1-liter bottle of extra virgin olive oil is over $3.50 on average. Can you imagine the oil savings you could get with an air fryer?

Lower consumption. Air fryers consume much less energy to prepare ingredients than conventional fryers. A point in favor of ecology and sustainable maintenance.

Chapter 1. Breakfast Recipes

1. Onion Frittata

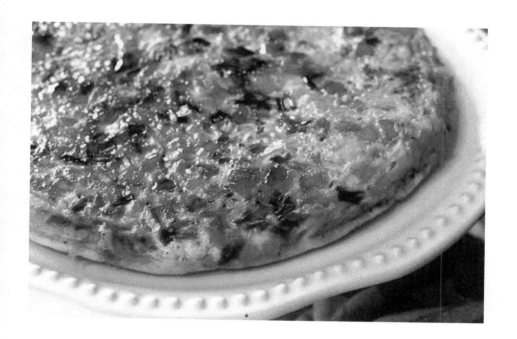

(Ready in about 30 min | Servings 6 | Easy)

Ingredients:

- 10 eggs, whisked

- 1 tablespoon of olive oil

- 1-pound of small potatoes, chopped

- 2 yellow onions, chopped

- Salt and black pepper to the taste

- 1-ounce of cheddar cheese, grated

- ½ cup sour cream

Directions:

1. Layer eggs with tomatoes, carrots, salt, pepper, cheese, and saucepan in a wide bowl and whisk well.

2. Grease the oil in the saucepan of your AirFryer, add the eggs, put in the AirFryer

And cook to 320° F for 20 minutes.

3. Slice the frittata, divide between the plates and serve as breakfast.

Enjoy!

Nutrition: Calories: 231, Fat: 5g, Fiber: 7g, Carbs: 8g, Protein: 4g.

2. Bell Peppers Frittata

(Ready in about 30 min | Servings 4 | Easy)

Ingredients:

- 2 tablespoons of olive oil

- ½ pounds of chicken sausage, casings removed and chopped

- 1 sweet onion, chopped

- 1 red bell pepper, chopped

- 1 orange bell pepper, chopped

- 1 green bell pepper, chopped

- Salt and black pepper to the taste

- 8 eggs, whisked

- ½ cup of mozzarella cheese, shredded

- 2 teaspoons of oregano, chopped

Directions:

1. Add 1 spoonful of oil to the AirFryer, add bacon, heat to 320° F, and brown for 1 minute.

2. Remove remaining butter, onion, red bell pepper, orange and white, mix and simmer for another 2 minutes.

3. Stir and cook for 15 minutes; add oregano, salt, pepper, and eggs.

4. Add mozzarella, leave frittata aside for a couple of minutes, divide and serve between plates.

Enjoy!

Nutrition: Calories: 212, Fat: 4g, Fiber: 6g, Carbs: 8g, Protein: 12g.

3. Cheese Sandwich

(Ready in about 18 min | Servings 1 | Easy)

Ingredients:

- 2 bread slices

- 2 teaspoons of butter

- 2 pieces of cheddar cheese

- A pinch of sweet paprika

Directions:

1. Place the butter on slices of bread, add the cheddar cheese on one, sprinkle the paprika, cover with the other slices of bread, break into 2 halves, put them in the AirFryer, and cook for 8 minutes at 370° F, turn them once, put them on a plate and serve.

Enjoy!

Nutrition: Calories: 130, Fat: 3g, Fiber: 5g, Carbs: 9g, Protein: 3g

4. Long Beans Omelet

(Ready in about 20 min | Servings 3 | Easy)

Ingredients:

- ½ teaspoon of soy sauce

- 1 tablespoon of olive oil

- 3 eggs, whisked

- A pinch of salt and black pepper

- 4 garlic cloves, minced

- 4 long beans, trimmed and sliced

Directions:

1. Mix the eggs in a bowl with a touch of salt, black pepper, and soy sauce, then whisk well.

4. At 320° F, fire up your AirFryer, add oil and garlic, stir, and brown for 1 minute.

3. Combine long beans and eggs, sprinkle and simmer for 10 minutes.

4. Break omelet into plates and serve for breakfast.

Enjoy!

Nutrition: Calories: 200, Fat: 3g, Fiber: 7g, Carbs: 9g, Protein: 3g.

5. French Beans and Egg Breakfast Mix

(Ready in about 20 min | Servings 3 | Easy)

Ingredients:

- 2 eggs, whisked

- ½ teaspoon of soy sauce

- 1 tablespoon of olive oil

- 4 garlic cloves, minced

- 3 ounces of French beans, trimmed and sliced diagonally

- Salt and white pepper to the taste

Directions:

1. Mix the eggs with soy sauce, salt, and pepper in a cup, then whisk properly.

2. Power the AirFryer up to 320° F, add oil, and fire it up too.

3. Add garlic and brown for 1 minute.

4. Remove French beans and egg mixture, toss for 10 minutes, then fry.

5. Serve for breakfast and split between dishes.

Enjoy!

Nutrition: Calories: 182, Fat: 3g, Fiber: 6g, Carbs: 8g, Protein: 3g.

Chapter 2. Sides, Snacks and Appetizers Recipes

6. Sausage Balls

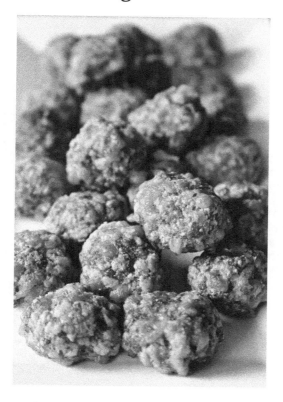

(Ready in about 25 min | Servings 9 | Normal)

Ingredients:

- 4 ounces of sausage meat, ground

- Salt and black pepper to the taste

- 1 teaspoon of sage

- ½ teaspoon of garlic, minced

- 1 small onion, chopped

- 3 tablespoons of breadcrumbs

Directions:

1. In a bowl, mix sausage with salt, pepper, sage, garlic, onion, and breadcrumbs, stir well and shape small balls out of this mix.

2. Put them in your AirFryer's basket, cook at 360° F for 15 minutes, divide into bowls and serve as a snack.

Enjoy!

Nutrition: Calories: 130, Fat: 7g, Fiber: 1g, Carbs: 13g, Protein: 4g.

7. Chicken Dip

(Ready in about 35 min | Servings 10 | Normal)

Ingredients:

- 3 tablespoons of butter, melted

- 1 cup of yogurt

- 12 ounces of cream cheese

- 2 cups of chicken meat, cooked and shredded

- 2 teaspoons of curry powder

- 4 scallions, chopped

- 6 ounces of Monterey jack cheese, grated

- 1/3 cup of raisins

- ¼ cup of cilantro, chopped

- ½ cup of almonds, sliced

- Salt and black pepper to the taste

- ½ cup of chutney

Directions:

1. In a bowl, mix cream cheese with yogurt and whisk using your mixer.

2. Add curry powder, scallions, chicken meat, raisins, cheese, cilantro, salt, and pepper and stir everything.

3. Spread this into a baking dish that fist your AirFryer, sprinkle almonds on top, place in your AirFryer, bake at 300° for 25 minutes, divide into bowls, top with chutney, and serve as an appetizer.

Enjoy!

Nutrition: Calories: 240, Fat: 10g, Fiber: 2g, Carbs: 24g, Protein: 12g.

8. Sweet Popcorn

(Ready in about 25 min | Servings 4 | Normal)

Ingredients:

- 2 tablespoons of corn kernels

- 2 and ½ tablespoons of butter

- 2 ounces of brown sugar

Directions:

1. Place the corn kernels in the pan of your AirFryer, cook them for 6 minutes at 400° F, move them to a plate, spread them out, and set them aside for now.

2. Heat a casserole over low pressure, add butter, melt it, add sugar, and whisk before dissolving.

3. Attach popcorn, throw to cover, heat off and scatter over the tray again.

4. Refrigerate, break into bowls, and serve as a snack.

Enjoy!

Nutrition: Calories: 70, Fat: 0.2g, Fiber: 0g, Carbs: 1g, Protein: 1g.

9. Apple Chips

(Ready in about 25 min | Servings 2 | Normal)

Ingredients:

- 1 apple, cored and sliced

- A pinch of salt

- ½ teaspoon of cinnamon powder

- 1 tablespoon of white sugar

Directions:

1. Mix apple slices with salt, sugar, and cinnamon in a cup, swirl, move to the basket from your AirFryer, cook at 390° F, tossing once for 10 minutes.

2. The apple chips are split into bowls and served as a snack.

Enjoy!

Nutrition: Calories: 70, Fat: 0g, Fiber: 4g, Carbs: 3g, Protein: 1g.

10. Bread Sticks

(Ready in about 20 min | Servings 2 | Normal)

Ingredients:

- 4 bread slices, each cut into 4 sticks

- 2 eggs

- ¼ cup of milk

- 1 teaspoon of cinnamon powder

- 1 tablespoon of honey

- ¼ cup of brown sugar

- A pinch of nutmeg

Directions:

1. In a cup, mix milk, brown sugar, cinnamon, nutmeg, and honey with the eggs and whisk well.

2. In this mix, dip the breadsticks, put them in the basket from your AirFryer, and cook for 10 minutes at 360° F.

3. Divide sticks of bread into bowls and serve as a snack.

Enjoy!

Nutrition: Calories: 140, Fat: 1g, Fiber: 4g, Carbs: 8g, Protein: 4g.

11. Crispy Shrimp

(Ready in about 15 min | Servings 4 | Normal)

Ingredients:

- 12 big shrimp, deveined and peeled

- 2 egg whites

- 1 cup of coconut, shredded

- 1 cup of panko bread crumbs

- 1 cup of white flour

- Salt and black pepper to the taste

Directions:

1. In a bowl, mix panko with coconut and stir.

2. Put flour, salt, and pepper in a second bowl and whisk egg whites in a third one.

3. Dip shrimp in flour, egg whites mix, and coconut, place them all in your AirFryer's basket, cook at 350° F for 10 minutes, flipping halfway.

4. Arrange on a platter and serve as an appetizer.

Enjoy!

Nutrition: Calories: 140, Fat: 4g, Fiber: 0g, Carbs: 3g, Protein: 4g.

12. Cajun Shrimp Appetizer

(Ready in about 15 min | Servings 2 | Normal)

Ingredients:

- 20 tiger shrimp, peeled and deveined

- Salt and black pepper to the taste

- ½ teaspoon of old bay seasoning

- 1 tablespoon of olive oil

- ¼ teaspoon of smoked paprika

Directions:

1. Mix shrimp and oil, salt, pepper, old bay seasoning, paprika in a dish, and mix to cover.

2. Place shrimp in the basket of your AirFryer and cook for 5 minutes at 390° F.

3. Put them up on a tray and act as an appetizer.

Enjoy!

Nutrition: Calories: 162, Fat: 6g, Fiber: 4g, Carbs: 8g, Protein: 14g.

13. Crispy Fish Sticks

(Ready in about 22 min | Servings 2 | Normal)

Ingredients:

- 4 ounces of bread crumbs

- 4 tablespoons of olive oil

- 1 egg, whisked

- 4 white fish filets, boneless, skinless, and cut into medium sticks

- Salt and black pepper to the taste

Directions:

1. Mix crumbs of bread with oil in a cup, then whisk well.

2. In a second tub, place the potato, apply the salt and pepper and whisk well.

3. Dip the fish stick in the egg, and the bread crumb mix, put them in the basket of your AirFryer, and cook for 12 minutes at 360° F.

4. Place fish sticks on a tray, and act as an appetizer.

Enjoy!

Nutrition: Calories: 160, Fat: 3g, Fiber: 5g, Carbs: 12g, Protein: 3g.

14. Fish Nuggets

(Ready in about 25 min | Servings 4 | Normal)

Ingredients:

- 28 ounces of fish fillets, skinless and cut into medium pieces

- Salt and black pepper to the taste

- 5 tablespoons of flour

- 1 egg, whisked

- 5 tablespoons of water

- 3 ounces of panko bread crumbs

- 1 tablespoon of garlic powder

- 1 tablespoon of smoked paprika

- 4 tablespoons of homemade mayonnaise

- Lemon juice from ½ lemon

- 1 teaspoon of dill, dried

- Cooking spray

Directions:

1. Mix the flour and water in a dish, then mix well.

2. Connect potato, pepper, and salt and whisk well.

3. Mix the panko with the garlic powder and paprika in a second dish, then stir well.

4. Sprinkle the pieces of fish in flour and egg mixture and then in panko mixture, put them in the basket of your AirFryer, spray them with the cooking oil and cook for 12 minutes at 400° F.

5. Meanwhile, blend dill and lemon juice mayo in a tub, and whisk well.

6. Arrange fish nuggets on a pan, then serve side by side with dill mayo.

Enjoy!

Nutrition: Calories: 332, Fat: 12g, Fiber: 6g, Carbs: 17g, Protein: 15g.

15. Shrimp and Chestnut Rolls

(Ready in about 25 min | Servings 4 | Normal)

Ingredients:

- ½ pound of already cooked shrimp, chopped

- 8 ounces of water chestnuts, chopped

- ½ pounds of shiitake mushrooms, chopped

- 2 cups of cabbage, chopped

- 2 tablespoons of olive oil

- 1 garlic clove, minced

- 1 teaspoon of ginger, grated

- 3 scallions, chopped

- Salt and black pepper to the taste

- 1 tablespoon of water

- 1 egg yolk

- 6 spring roll wrappers

Directions:

1. Heat a skillet over medium-high heat with the oil, add cabbage, shrimp, chestnuts, mushrooms, garlic, ginger, salt, and pepper, stir and simmer for 2 minutes.

2. Mix the egg and water in a dish, then combine well.

3. Arrange roll wrappers on a working board, slice shrimp and veggie mix into them, seal edges with egg wash, put them all in the basket of your AirFryer, cook for 15 minutes at 360° F, move to a plate, and serve as an appetizer.

Enjoy!

Nutrition: Calories: 140, Fat: 3g, Fiber: 1g, Carbs: 12g, Protein: 3g.

Chapter 3. Vegetable and Vegetarian Recipes

16. Balsamic Potatoes

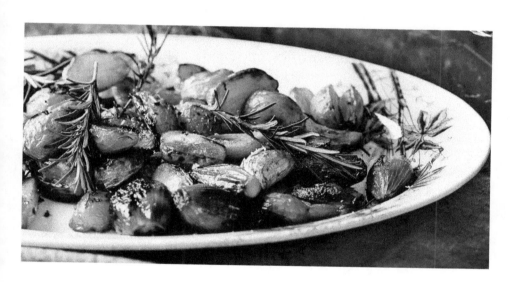

(Ready in about 30 min | Servings 4 | Easy)

Ingredients:

- 1 and ½ pounds of baby potatoes, halved

- 2 garlic cloves, chopped

- 2 red onions, chopped

- 9 ounces of cherry tomatoes

- 3 tablespoons of olive oil

- 1 and ½ tablespoons of balsamic vinegar

- 2 thyme springs, chopped

- Salt and black pepper to the taste

Directions:

1. Mix the garlic with the onions, oil, vinegar, thyme, salt, pepper, and pulse very well in your food processor.

2. Mix the tomatoes and the balsamic marinade in a cup, mix properly, move to your AirFryer and cook for 20 minutes at 380° F.

3. Divide between plates and eat.

Enjoy!

Nutrition: Calories: 301, Fat: 6g, Fiber: 8g, Carbs: 18g, Protein: 6g.

17. Potatoes and Special Tomato Sauce

(Ready in about 26 min | Servings 4 | Easy)

Ingredients:

- 2 pounds of potatoes, cubed

- 4 garlic cloves, minced

- 1 yellow onion, chopped

- 1 cup of tomato sauce

- 2 tablespoons of basil, chopped

- 2 tablespoons of olive oil

- ½ teaspoon of oregano, dried

- ½ teaspoon of parsley, dried

Directions:

1. Heat a saucepan over medium heat that matches your AirFryer with the oil, add onion, stir and cook for 1-2 minutes.

2. Add the garlic, cabbage, parsley, tomato sauce, and oregano, stir, place in the AirFryer and cook for 16 minutes at 370° F.

3. Add basil, mix it all, break into plates and eat.

Enjoy!

Nutrition: Calories: 211, Fat: 6g, Fiber: 8g, Carbs: 14g, Protein: 6g.

18. Loaded Cauliflower Steak

(Ready in about 14 min | Servings 4 | Easy)

Ingredients:

- 1 medium head cauliflower

- 1/4 cup of hot sauce

- 2 tablespoons of salted butter, melted

- 1/4 cup of blue cheese crumbles

- 1/4 cup of full-Fat: ranch dressing

Directions:

1. Cut the leaves of a cauliflower. Break the head into thick slices of ½.

2. Add the hot sauce and butter in a shallow dish. Rub the cauliflower mixture around it.

3. Put each steak of the cauliflower in the AirFryer and operate in batches where appropriate.

4. Set the temperature to 400° F and set the timer for seven minutes.

5. The edges may start becoming dark and caramelized when baked.

6. Brush on crumbled blue cheesesteaks to eat. Drizzle seasoning with grass.

Enjoy!

Nutrition: Calories: 122,Protein: 4.9g, Fiber: 3.0g, Net Carbohydrates: 4.7g, Fat: 8.4g,Sodium: 283 mg, Carbohydrates: 7.7g sugar: 2.9g.

19. Three-Cheese Zucchini Boats

(Ready in about 35 min | Servings 2 | Normal)

Ingredients:

- 2 medium zucchinis

- 1 tablespoon of avocado oil

- 1/4 cup of low-carb, no-sugar-added pasta sauce

- 1/4 cup of full-Fat: ricotta cheese

- 1/4 cup of shredded mozzarella cheese

- 1/4 teaspoon of dried oregano

- 1/4 teaspoon of garlic powder

- 1/2 teaspoon of dried parsley

- 2 tablespoons grated vegetarian Parmesan cheese

- 1 zucchini, cut off 1" from the top and bottom.

Directions:

1. Slice the zucchini in half lengthwise and use a spoon to scrape out a little bit of the cavity, allowing room for fill. Clean 2 spoonful of pasta sauce with oil and spoon into each cup.

2. Mix ricotta, mozzarella, oregano, garlic powder, and parsley in a medium saucepan. Spoon the mixture into the shell of each zucchini. Place packed courgettes into shells

3. Set the temperature to 350° F and change the timer for 20 minutes.

4. Use tongs or a spatula to detach from the fryer bowl and hold it carefully. Strong on Parmesan.

Serve immediately.

Nutrition: Calories: 215, Protein: 10.5g, Fiber: 2.7g, Net Carbohydrates: 6.6g Fat: 14.9g, Sodium: 386 mg, Carbohydrates: 9.3g sugar: 5.2g.

20. Portobello Mini Pizzas

(Ready in about 20 min | Servings 4 | Normal)

Ingredients:

- 2 large portobello mushrooms

- 2 tablespoons of unsalted butter, melted

- 1/2 teaspoon of garlic powder

- 2/3 cup of shredded mozzarella cheese

- 4 grape tomatoes, sliced

- 2 leaves of fresh basil, chopped

- 1 tablespoon of balsamic vinegar

Directions:

1. Excavate the interior of the mushrooms and leave only the tips. Put butter on each cap and sprinkle with the garlic powder.

2. Fill each cap with the sliced tomatoes and the mozzarella. Place each mini pizza in a 6" round

baking pan. Put the pan into the basket with the AirFryer.

3. Set the temperature to 380° F and set the timer for a further 10 minutes.

4. Extract the pizzas from the fryer basket slowly and garnish them with basil and vinegar.

Nutrition: Calories: 244, Protein: 10.4g, Fiber: 1.4g, Net Carbohydrates 5.4g Fat: 18.5g, Sodium: 244 mg, Carbohydrates 6.8g sugar 4.3g.

21. Veggie Quesadilla

(Ready in about 15 min | Servings 2 | Easy)

Ingredients:

- 1 tablespoon of coconut oil

- 1/2 medium green bell pepper, seeded and chopped

- 1/4 cup of diced red onion

- 1/4 cup chopped of white mushrooms

- 4 flatbread dough tortillas

- 2/3 cup of shredded pepper jack cheese

- 1/2 medium avocado, peeled, pitted, and mashed

- 1/4 cup of full-Fat: sour cream

- 1/4 cup of mild salsa

Directions:

1. Warm coconut oil in a medium saucepan over low pressure. Add pepper, onion, and mushrooms to skillet and sauté for 3–5 minutes before peppers begin to soften.

2. Put two tortillas on a work surface and sprinkle half the cheese on each. Cover with sautéed onions, scatter with remaining cheese, and finish with two tortillas left. Carefully put quesadillas inside the bowl of the AirFryer.

3. Change the temperature to 400° F and set a 5-minute timer.

4. Flip the quesadillas halfway through the cycle of preparation. Serve mild with avocado and sour cream, along with salsa.

Nutrition: Calories: 795,Protein: 34.5g,Fiber: 6.5g,Net Carbohydrates 12.9g Fat: 61.3g, Sodium 1,051 mg, Carbohydrates: 19.4g sugar: 7.4g.

22. Alternative Tortillas

(Ready in about 25 min | Servings 2 | Normal)

Ingredients:

- 1 cup of broccoli florets

- 1 cup of quartered Brussels sprouts

- 1/2 cup of cauliflower florets

- 1/4 medium white onion, peeled and sliced

- 1/4" thick 1/2 medium green bell pepper, seeded and sliced

- 1 tablespoon of coconut oil

- 2 teaspoons of chili powder

- 1/2 teaspoon of garlic powder

- 1/2 teaspoon of cumin

Directions:

1. In a wide tub, mix all ingredients until the vegetables are thoroughly covered with oil and seasoning.

2. Verse the vegetables into the tray of the AirFryer.

3. Set the temperature to 360° F and change the timer for 15 minutes.

4. When cooking, shake two to three times. Serve and enjoy.

Nutrition: Calories: 121,Protein: 4.3g,Fiber: 5.2g,Net Carbohydrates: 7.9g Fat: 7.1 g,Sodium: 112 mg, Carbohydrates: 13.1 g sugar: 3.8g.

23. Spinach Artichoke Casserole

(Ready in about 30 min | Servings 4 | Easy)

Ingredients:

- 1 tablespoon of salted butter, melted

- 1/4 cup of diced yellow onion

- 8 ounces of full-Fat: cream cheese, softened

- 1/3 cup of full-Fat: mayonnaise

- 1/3 cup of full-Fat: sour cream

- 1/4 cup of chopped pickled jalapeños

- 2 cups of fresh spinach, chopped

- 2 cups of cauliflower florets, chopped

- 1 cup of artichoke hearts, chopped

Directions:

1. Add butter, onion, cream cheese, mayonnaise, and sour cream in a big cup. Jalapeños, lettuce, cauliflower, and artichokes fold in.

2. Pour the mixture into a circular baking dish with 4 cups. Cover with tape, and put in the basket of the AirFryer.

3. Set the temperature to 370° F and change the timer for 15 minutes.

4. Cut foil over the last 2 minutes of cooking to brown the end. Serve and enjoy.

Nutrition: Calories: 423, Protein: 6.7g, Fiber: 5.3g, Net Carbohydrates: 6.8g, Fat: 36.3g, Sodium: 495 mg, Carbohydrates: 12.1g sugar: 4.4g.

Chapter 4. Pork, Beef, and Lamb Recipes

24. Mustard Beef Ted at Marina

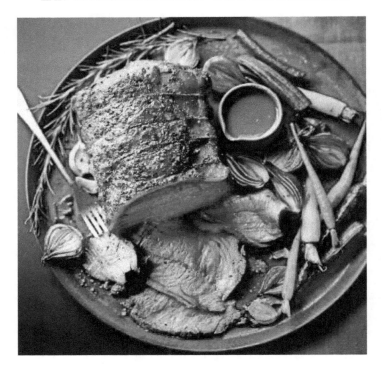

(Ready in about 55 min | Servings 6 | Normal)

Ingredients:

- Six strips of bacon

- Two cups of butter

- Three cloves of garlic, diced

- Salt and black pepper, to the taste

- One spoonful of horseradish

- One tsp of mustard

- Three lbs. of roast beef

- One and 3/4 cup stocks of beef

- Red 3/4 cup wine

Directions:

1. In a bowl, combine butter, garlic, salt, pepper, and mustard. This mixture includes horseradish, whisk, and rub beef.

2. Place bacon strips on a cutting board, put the beef on top, fold bacon with the meat, switch to the basket of your AirFryer, cook at 400° F for fifteen min, then switch to a fryer-fitting pan.

3. Add stock and wine to the beef, put the saucepan in the AirFryer, and cook thirty min higher at 360° Fahrenheit.

4. Carve the beef, break between plates, and share with a side salad.

Enjoy!

Nutrition: Calories: 500, Fat: 9g, Fiber: 4g, Carbohydrates 29g, Protein: 36g.

25. Garlic Mayo Beef Fillets

(Ready in about 50 min | Servings 8 | Normal)

Ingredients:

- One slice of mayonnaise

- 1/3 teaspoons of sour cream

- Two cloves of garlic, minced

- Three lb. of beef fillet

- Two spoonfuls of chives, chopped

- Two mustard spoons

- Two mustard spoons

- 1/4 cup estragon, split

- Salt and black chili, to try

Directions:

1. Season the beef to taste with salt and pepper, put in the AirFryer, cook for 20 minutes at 370 °F,

switch to a saucepan, and have a few minutes left-back.

2. Blend the garlic in a bowl of sour cream, mustard, mayo, a few salt, pepper, whisk, and withdraw.

3. Blend the mustard with Dijon mustard and tarragon in another dish, whisk, add beef, shake, transfer to the frying pan, and cook for twenty minutes more° 350 F.

4. Split the beef into bowls, sprinkle the mayo with garlic over them, and eat.

Enjoy!

Nutrition: Calories: 400, Fat: 12g, Fiber: 2g, Carbohydrates 27g, Protein: 19g.

26. Brussels Lamb and Fluffy Sprouts

(Ready in about 1hr 20 min | Servings 4 | Difficult)

Ingredients:

- Two lbs leg of lamb scored

- Two lbs. of olive oil

- One spoonful of rosemary, chopped

- 1 liter of lemon thyme, diced

- One clove of garlic, minced

- Brussels sprouts, one and 1/2 pounds, trimmed

- One tablespoon butter, warmed

- 1/2 cup of sour cream

- Salt and black pepper, to satisfy

Directions:

1. Season lamb leg with salt, pepper, thyme, and rosemary, pinch, and cook with oil, put in the basket of your AirFryer, 300° F for 1 hour. Switch to a plate, and stay wet.

2. Mix the Brussels sprouts with salt in a saucepan that suits your AirFryer, toss the tomato, ginger, butter, and sour cream, put the fryer in your air, and cook for 10 minutes, at 400° Fahrenheit

3. Split the lamb into bowls, place the sprouts on the side and eat.

Enjoy!

Nutrition: Calories: 440, Fat: 23g, Fiber: 0, Carbohydrates 2g, Protein: 49g.

27. Indian Pork

(Ready in about 45 min | Servings 4 | Normal)

Ingredients:

- One teaspoon of ground ginger

- 2 tsp of chili paste

- Two cloves of garlic, minced

- Fourteen ounces of pork chops, wrapped in cubes

- One shallot, cut

- One coriander with a teaspoon, ground

- Seven ounces of coconut milk

- 2 tsp of olive oil

- Three ounces of peanuts, planet

- Three spoonfuls of soy sauce

- Salt and black chili, to try

Directions:

1. Place the ginger and 1 teaspoon of chili paste in a cup, half the garlic, half the soy sauce, and quarter the grease, shake, introduce the meat, and mix. Put on for ten min.

2. Switch meat to the basket of your AirFryer and cook 400° F. Switch midway, for 12 minutes.

3. In the meantime, fire up a pan over medium-high heat with the rest of the oil, add shallot, remaining garlic, coriander, coconut milk, the remaining peas, the remaining chili paste, and the majority of the soy. Stir in the gravy, and simmer for five min.

4. Start dividing pork into bowls, place coconut mixture above, and eat.

Enjoy!

Nutrition: Calories: 423, Fat: 11g, fruit 4g, Carbohydrates 42g, Protein: 18g.

28. Crystal Lamb

(Ready in about 40 min | Servings 4 | Normal)

Ingredients:

- 1 tsp of bread crumbs

- Two tablespoons of macadamia nuts, roasted and toasted

- 1 tsp of olive oil

- One clove of garlic, diced

- 28 ounces of lamb rack

- Salt and black chili, to the taste

- 1 egg

- One spoonful of rosemary, chopped

Directions:

1. Blend the oil and garlic in a cup, then stir well.

2. Dress lamb to the oil with salt, pepper, and brush.

3. Place the nuts with the breadcrumbs and rosemary into another dish.

4. Place the egg in a different saucepan and stir well.

5. Soak the lamb in the milk, then blend it in the macadamia, put it in your air heat basket with fryer at 360 °F, and steam for 25 minutes. Heat up to 400° F, and simmer for another five min.

6. Split between bowls, and serve immediately.

Enjoy!

Nutrition: Calories: 230, Fat: 2g, Carbohydrates 10g, Protein: 12g.

29. Chops the Garlic Lamb

(Ready in about 20 min | Servings 4 | Normal)

Ingredients:

- Three tsp of olive oil

- Eight lamb chops

- Salt and black chili, to satisfy

- Four cloves of garlic, diced

- One spoonful of oregano, sliced

- One tsp of coriander, diced

Directions:

1. Comb the oregano in a bowl of salt, pepper, milk, garlic, chopped lamb, and shake.

2. Switch the chopped lamb to the fryer and prepare at 400 °F for just ten minutes.

3. On bowls, split the lamb chops and start serving with a side salad.

Enjoy it!

Nutrition: Calories: 231, Fat: 7g, Fiber: 5g, Carbohydrates 14g, Protein: 23g.

Chapter 5. Fish and Sea Food

30. Fillet Cod and Peas

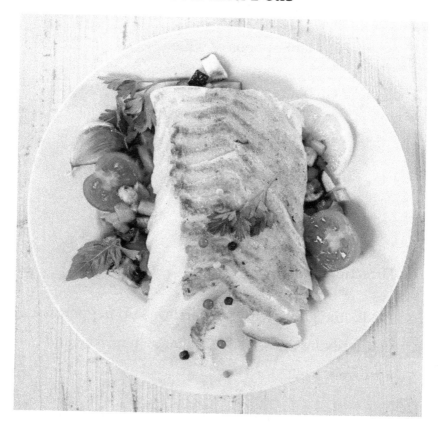

(Ready in about 20 min | Servings 4 | Normal)

Ingredients:

- 4 cod fillets, boneless

- 2 tablespoons of parsley, chopped

- Two cups of peas

- Four tablespoons of wine

- 2 tsp of oregano, dry

- 1/2 cup of tender paprika

- Two cloves of garlic, minced

- Salt and chili to try

Directions:

1. Mix the garlic with the parsley, salt, pepper in your mixing bowl, add oregano, paprika, and juice, mix well.

2. Rub the fish with half of this combination, put the fryer in the air, and cook for 10 minutes at 360° F.

3. In the meantime, place the peas in a kettle, add water to cover, add salt and bring to boil over medium pressure, simmer for ten minutes. Divide into plates.

4. Divide fish into bowls, scatter the rest of the herb dressing over and serve.

Enjoy it!

Nutrition: Calories: 261, Fat: 8g, Fiber: 12g, Carbohydrates 20g, Protein: 22g.

31. Fillet Truffle and Orange Sauce

(Ready in about 20 min | Servings 4 | Normal)

Ingredients:

- Four fillets of trout, skinless and boneless

- Four onions in the spring, minced

- 1 tablespoon of olive oil

- 1 tablespoon of ginger, minced

- Salt and black chili, to try

- 1 orange juice and zest

Directions:

1. Season the fillets with salt and pepper, rub them with the oil, put in a saucepan that suits your fryer, add the ginger, the green onions, orange zest, and juice, stir well, placed in the fryer, and cook for 10 minutes at 360° F.

2. Divide fish and sauce into bowls and serve immediately.

Enjoy!

Nutrition: Calories: 239, Fat: 10g, Fiber: 7g, Carbohydrates 18g, Protein: 23g.

32. Casserole Seafood

(Ready in about 50 min | Servings 6 | Normal)

Ingredients:

- Six tablespoons of butter

- Two ounces of champignons, chopped

- One little green bell pepper chopped

- One stalk of celery hacked

- Two cloves of garlic, minced

- 1 small yellow, diced onion

- Salt and black chili, to try

- Four teaspoons of flour

- White wine: 1/2 cup

- 1 and a half cups of milk

- 4 Scallops at sea, cut

- 4 ounces of haddock, skinless, boneless and cut into small parts

- 4 ounces of lobster meat already cooked and cut into small pieces

- 1/2 teaspoon of mustard powder

- 1 tablespoon of lemon juice

- 1/3 cup of crumbs of bread

- Salt and black chili, to try

- 3 spoonful of cheddar cheese, grated

- A tablespoon of sliced parsley

- 1 teaspoon of sweet paprika

Directions:

1. Heat a saucepan with 4 spoons butter over medium pressure, whisk in bell pepper, chestnuts, celery, garlic, onion, and wine. Then, boil for ten minutes.

2. Stir well and simmer for 6 minutes. Add flour, cream, and milk.

3. Add lemon juice, salt, pepper, ground mustard, scallops, lobster, meat, and haddock, stir well, heat off, and transfer to a saucepan that fits the fryer.

4. Mix the remaining butter in a dish with the breadcrumbs, paprika, and sprinkle with cheese over the seafood mixture.

5. Switch the saucepan to the AirFryer and cook at 360° F for 16 minutes.

6. Divide between bowls, then serve sprinkled on top of parsley.

Enjoy!

Nutrition: Calories: 270, Fat: 32g, Fiber: 14g, Carbohydrates 15g, Protein: 23g.

33. Shrimp and Mix with Crab

(Ready in about 35 min | Servings 4 | Normal)

Ingredients:

- 1/2 cup of yellow, minced onion

- 1 cup of green potatoes, diced

- 1 cup of celery, cut

- 1 pound of crawls, sliced

- 1 cup of crabmeat, sliced

- 1 cup of mayonnaise

- 1 Worcestershire teaspoon sauce

- Salt and black chili, to try

- 2 tablespoons of sliced bread

- 1 tablespoon of butter, melted

- 1 tablespoon of tender paprika

Directions:

1. Comb shrimp and crab meat in a dish, bell pepper, tomato, mayo, sauce with celery, garlic, chili pepper, and Worcestershire, mix well and pass to the casserole that suits your fryer.

2. Sprinkle the crumbs and the paprika with the crust, apply the melted butter and put in

your AirFryer and bake for 25 minutes at 320° F, midway.

3. Divide between bowls and serve immediately.

Enjoy!

Nutrition: Calories: 200, Fat: 13g, Fiber: 9g, Carbohydrates 17g, Protein: 19g.

34. Cod and Vinaigrette

(Ready in about 25 min | Servings 4 | Normal)

Ingredients:

- Four cod fillets, skinless and boneless

- 12 halved cherry tomatoes

- 8 black olives, finely chopped and pitted

- 2 tablespoons of lemon juice

- Salt and black chili, to try

- 2 tablespoons of olive oil

- Cooking spray

- 1 packet of basil, chopped

Directions:

1. Season cod with salt and pepper to taste, put in the AirFryers bucket, and cook for 10 minutes at 360° F for five minutes.

2. In the meantime, prepare a saucepan over medium heat with the oil, add the onions, olives, and lemon juice, bring to a boil, add basil. Stir well with salt and pepper, and take off fire.

3. Segregate fish into plates and serve on top with the drizzled vinaigrette.

Enjoy!

Nutrition: Calories: 300, Fat: 5g, Fiber: 8g, Carbohydrates 12g, Protein: 8g.

Chapter 6. Poultry Recipes

35. Creamy Coconut Chicken

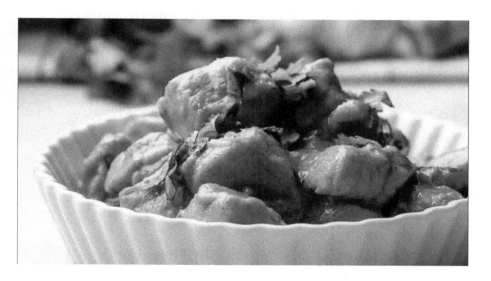

(Ready in about 2hr 25 min | Servings 4 | Difficult)

Ingredients:

- 4 big chicken legs

- 5 teaspoons of turmeric powder

- 2 tablespoons of ginger, grated

- Salt and black pepper to the taste

- 4 tablespoons of coconut cream

Directions:

1. In a bowl, mix the cream with turmeric, ginger, salt, and pepper, whisk, add chicken pieces, toss them well and leave aside for 2 hours.

2. Transfer chicken to your preheated AirFryer, cook at 370° F for 25 minutes, divide among plates and serve with a side salad.

Enjoy!

Nutrition: Calories: 300, Fat: 4g, Fiber: 12g, Carbs: 22g, Protein: 20g.

36. Chinese Chicken Wings

(Ready in about 2hr 15 min | Servings 6 | Normal)

Ingredients:

- 16 chicken wings

- 2 tablespoons of honey

- 2 tablespoons of soy sauce

- Salt and black pepper to the taste

- ¼ teaspoon of white pepper

- 3 tablespoons of lime juice

Directions:

1. In a bowl, mix honey with soy sauce, salt, black and white pepper, and lime juice, whisk well, add chicken pieces, toss to coat and keep in the fridge for 2 hours.

2. Transfer chicken to your AirFryer, cook at 370° F for 6 minutes on each side, increase heat to 400° F and cook for 3 minutes more.

3. Serve hot.

Enjoy!

Nutrition: Calories: 372, Fat: 9g, Fiber: 10g, Carbs: 37g, Protein: 24g.

37. Herbed Chicken

(Ready in about 1hr 10 min | Servings 4 | Difficult)

Ingredients:

- 1 whole chicken

- Salt and black pepper to the taste

- 1 teaspoon of garlic powder

- 1 teaspoon of onion powder

- ½ teaspoon of thyme, dried

- 1 teaspoon of rosemary, dried

- 1 tablespoon of lemon juice

- 2 tablespoons of olive oil

Directions:

1. Season chicken with salt and pepper, rub with thyme, rosemary, garlic powder, and onion

powder, rub with lemon juice and olive oil and leave aside for 30 minutes.

2. Put the chicken in your AirFryer and cook at 360° F for 20 minutes on each side.

3. Leave chicken aside to cool down, carve and serve.

Enjoy!

Nutrition: Calories: 390, Fat: 10g, Fiber: 5g, Carbs: 22g, Protein: 20g.

38. Chicken Parmesan

(Ready in about 25 min | Servings 4 | Normal)

Ingredients:

- 2 cups of panko bread crumbs

- ¼ cup of parmesan, grated

- ½ teaspoon of garlic powder

- 2 cups of white flour

- 1 egg, whisked

- 1 and ½ pounds of chicken cutlets, skinless and boneless

- Salt and black pepper to the taste

- 1 cup of mozzarella, grated

- 2 cups of tomato sauce

- 3 tablespoons of basil, chopped

Directions:

1. In a bowl, mix panko with parmesan and garlic powder and stir.

2. Put flour in a second bowl and the egg in a third.

3. Season chicken with salt and pepper, dip in flour, then in the egg mix, and panko.

4. Put chicken pieces in your AirFryer and cook them at 360° F for 3 minutes on each side.

5. Transfer chicken to a baking dish that fits your AirFryer, add tomato sauce and top with mozzarella, introduce in your AirFryer and cook at 375° F for 7 minutes.

6. Divide among plates, sprinkle basil on top, and serve.

Enjoy!

Nutrition: Calories: 304, Fat: 12g, Fiber: 11g, Carbs: 22g, Protein: 15g.

39. Mexican Chicken

(Ready in about 30 min | Servings 4 | Normal)

Ingredients:

- 16 ounces of green salsa

- 1 tablespoon of olive oil

- Salt and black pepper to the taste

- 1 pound of chicken breast, boneless and skinless

- 1 and ½ cup of Monterey Jack cheese, grated

- ¼ cup of cilantro, chopped

- 1 teaspoon of garlic powder

Directions:

1. Pour green salsa in a baking dish that fits your AirFryer, season chicken with salt, pepper, garlic

powder, brush with olive oil and place it over your green salsa.

2. Introduce in your AirFryer and cook at 380° F for 20 minutes.

3. Sprinkle cheese on top and cook for 2 minutes more.

4. Divide among plates and serve hot.

Enjoy!

Nutrition: Calories: 340, Fat: 18g, Fiber: 14g, Carbs: 32g, Protein: 18g.

40. Creamy Chicken, Rice, and Peas

(Ready in about 40 min | Servings 4 | Normal)

Ingredients:

- 1 pound of chicken breasts, skinless, boneless, and cut into quarters

- 1 cup of white rice, already cooked

- Salt and black pepper to the taste

- 1 tablespoon of olive oil

- 3 garlic cloves, minced

- 1 yellow onion, chopped

- ½ cup of white wine

- ¼ cup of heavy cream

- 1 cup of chicken stock

- ¼ cup of parsley, chopped

- 2 cups of peas, frozen

- 1 and ½ cups of parmesan, grated

Directions:

1. Season chicken breasts with salt and pepper, drizzle half of the oil over them, rub well, put in your AirFryer's basket, and cook them at 360° F for 6 minutes.

2. Heat a pan with the rest of the oil over medium-high heat, add garlic, onion, wine, stock, salt, pepper, and heavy cream, stir, bring to a simmer and cook for 9 minutes.

3. Transfer chicken breasts to a heatproof dish that fits your AirFryer, add peas, rice, and cream mix over them, toss, sprinkle parmesan, and parsley all over, place in your AirFryer and cook at 420° F for 10 minutes.

4. Divide among plates and serve hot.

Enjoy!

Nutrition: Calories: 313, Fat: 12g, Fiber: 14g, Carbs: 27g, Protein: 44g.

Chapter 7. Desserts and Sweets Recipes

41. Asian Halibut

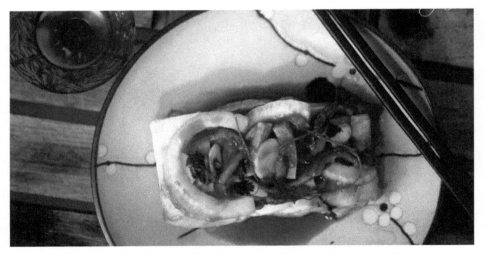

(Ready in about 40 min | Servings 3 | Normal)

Ingredients:

- 1 lb of halibut steaks

- Soy sauce: 2/3 cup

- One and a half cup of sugar

- 2 spoonful of lime juice

- 1/2 cup of mirin

- 1/4 teaspoon red pepper flakes

- 1/4 tablespoon of orange juice

- 1/4 tablespoon of ginger powder, grated

- 1 clove of garlic, minced

Directions:

1. Place soy sauce in a saucepan, fire over a moderate flame, including mirin, sugar, lime and orange juice, ginger and garlic, pepper flakes, blend well. Bring it to a boil, and heat off.

2. Put half of the marinade in a cup, add halibut, toss to cover, then leave them in the refrigerator for 30 minutes.

3. Switch the halibut to the AirFryer and cook for 10 minutes at 390° F, only flipping once.

4. Divide halibut steaks into bowls, scatter with the rest of the marinade. Serve and enjoy!

Nutrition: Calories: 286, Fat: 5g, Fiber: 12g, Carbohydrates 14g, Protein: 23g.

42. Marine Lemon Saba

(Ready in about 18 min | Servings 1 | Normal)

Ingredients:

- 4 Sheba fish fillets

- Salt and black chili, to satisfy

- 3 red peppered chilies, minced

- 2 tablespoons of lemon juice

- 2 1/2 cubit of olive oil

- 2 teaspoons of garlic, chopped

Directions:

1. Season fish fillets and placed in a bowl of salt and pepper.

2. Add lemon juice, milk, chili, and garlic to coat, and pass to the freezer the air and cook for 8 minutes at 360° F, midway.

3. Divide between bowls and serve with a few fries.

Enjoy it!

Nutrition: Calories: 300, Fat: 4g, Fiber: 8g, Carbohydrates 15g, Protein: 15g.

43. Salmon with Capers and Mash

(Ready in about 30 min | Servings 4 | Normal)

Ingredients:

- 4 skinless and boneless salmon fillets

- 1 spoonful of caper, drained

- Salt and black chili, to try

- 1 lemon juice

- 2 cups of olive oil

For mash potatoes:

- 2 tablespoons of olive oil

- 1 tablespoon of dill, dry

- 1 pound of diced potatoes

- 1/2 cup of milk

Directions:

1. Place the potatoes in a saucepan, add a little water, add some salt, bring to boil over a moderate flame, cook for fifteen min, drain, switch to low heat. In a bowl, pound with a potato masher, add 2 cubic cubes of oil, dill, honey, and whisk the pepper and milk good, and set aside for now.

2. Season salmon with salt and pepper and drizzle oil over 2 teaspoons, them, rub, transfer to your AirFryer's basket, add capers on top. Cook for 8 minutes, at 360° F.

3. Break salmon and capers into bowls, add mashed potatoes to the pan, drizzle the lemon juice over the side and eat.

Enjoy!

Nutrition: Calories: 300, Fat: 17g, Fiber: 8g, Carbohydrates 12g, Protein: 18g.

44. Aromatized Air Fried Salmon

(Ready in about 1hr 8 min | Servings 2 | Normal)

Ingredients:

- Two salmon fillets

- Two tablespoons of lemon juice

- Salt and black chili, to try

- 1/2 teaspoon crushed garlic

- 1/3 cup of soy sauce

- 3 chopped scallions

- 1/3 cup of brown sugar

- 2 tablespoons of olive oil

Directions:

1. In a cup, add water to the sugar, soy sauce, garlic powder, salt. Sprinkle with vinegar, oil, and lemon juice, whisk well, add salmon fillets and toss. Cover in the fridge and set aside for 1 hour.

2. Move the salmon fillets into the fryer's basket and cook at 360° F, flipping them in half for 8 minutes.

3. Divide the salmon into bowls, scatter the scallions on top and serve appropriately.

Enjoy it!

Nutrition: Calories: 300, Fat: 12g, Fiber: 10g, Carbohydrates 23g, Protein: 20g.

45. Steaks Cod with Plum Sauce

(Ready in about 30 min | Servings 2 | Normal)

Ingredients:

- 2 big cod steaks

- Salt and black chili, to satisfy

- 1/2 teaspoon crushed garlic

- 1/2 cubicle ginger powder

- 1/4 tablespoon of turmeric powder

- 1 tablespoon of plum sauce

- Cooking spray

Directions:

1. Season cod steaks with salt and pepper, sprinkle with cream, apply powdered garlic, ginger powder, and turmeric powder, and rub well.

2. Place cod steaks in your AirFryer and cook for 15 Minutes at 360° F, after 7 minutes.

3. Heat a casserole over medium heat, add prune sauce, stir and cook for just 2 minutes.

4. Divide the cod steaks into bowls, drizzle all over the plum sauce and serve.

Enjoy!

Nutrition: 250 Calories:, Fat: 7, Fiber: 1, 14 Carbohydrates, 12g Protein:.

46. Asian Salmon

(Ready in about 1hr 15 min | Servings 2 | Normal)

Ingredients:

- 2 moderate fillet salmon

- Six spoonsful of medium soy sauce

- Three mirin teaspoons

- 1 tablespoon of water

- Six honey spoons

Directions:

1. Mix the soy sauce and sugar, water, and mirin in a container, shake well. Bring salmon, rub well, and put in the refrigerator for 1 hour.

2. Transfer the salmon to the AirFryer and cook for 15 minutes, at 360° F; after 7 minutes, flip.

3. Put the soy marinade in a saucepan, flame over medium heat up, whisk properly, simmer for 2 minutes, and turn off.

4. Break salmon on bowls, chop marinade all over, and eat.

Enjoy!

Nutrition: Calories: 300, Fat: 12g, Fiber: 8g, Carbohydrates 13g, Protein: 24g.

47. Buttered Shrimp Skewers

(Ready in about 16 min | Servings 2 | Normal)

Ingredients:

- Eight shrimps, sliced

- Four cloves of garlic, diced

- Salt and black chili, to try

- Eight slices of green bell pepper

- 1 spoonful of rosemary, chopped

- 1 tablespoon of butter, melted

Directions:

1. Mix the shrimp with the garlic, butter, salt, pepper, rosemary in a dish, and slices of pepper bell, swirl to cover, and keep on for ten minutes.

2. Put 2 shrimp and 2 slices of bell pepper on a skewer and repeat for the remaining bits of shrimp and bell pepper.

3. Place all in the basket of your AirFryer and cook 360° F for six minutes.

4. Segregate between bowls, and serve immediately.

Enjoy!

Nutrition: Calories: 140, Fat: 1g, Fiber: 12g, Carbohydrates 15g, Protein: 7g.

48. Shrimp Tabasco

(Ready in about 20 min | Servings 4 | Normal)

Ingredients:

- 1 pound of shrimps, sliced

- 1 teaspoon red pepper flakes

- Two tablespoons of olive oil

- 1 Tabasco teaspoon sauce

- 2 cups of water

- 1 tsp of dried oregano

- Salt and black chili, to try

- 1/2 teaspoon of dried parsley

- 1/2 smoked paprika teaspoon

Directions:

1. Mix oil and water in a tub, Tabasco sauce, pepper flakes, oregano, parsley, rice, vinegar, bell pepper, shrimp, and mix well.

2. Transfer shrimps to 370° F to your hot oven AirFryer and cook, turning the fryer once for ten minutes.

3. On bowls, split the shrimp and serve with a side salad.

Enjoy it!

Nutrition: 200 Calories:, 5 Fat:, 6 Fiber:, 13 Carbohydrates, 8g Protein:.

Chapter 8. Lunch Recipes

49. Lunch Special Pancake

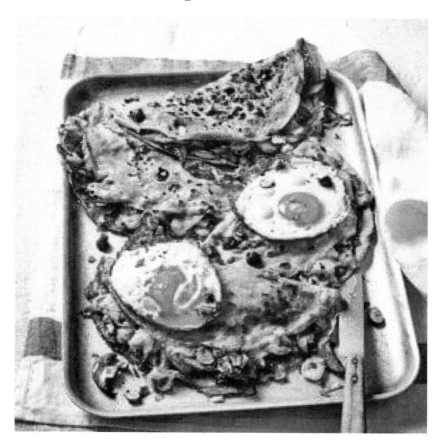

(Ready in about 20 min | Servings 2 | Normal)

Ingredients:

- 1 tablespoon of butter

- 3 eggs, whisked

- ½ cup of flour

- ½ cup of milk

- 1 cup of salsa

- 1 cup of small shrimp, peeled and deveined

Directions:

1. Preheat your AirFryer at 400° F, add fryer's pan, add 1 tablespoon butter, and melt it.

2. In a bowl, mix eggs with flour and milk, whisk well, and pour into the AirFryer's pan, spread, cook at 350° for 12 minutes, and transfer to a plate.

3. In a bowl, mix shrimp with salsa, stir and serve your pancake with this on the side.

Enjoy!

Nutrition: Calories: 200, Fat: 6g, Fiber: 8g, Carbs: 12g, Protein: 4g.

50. Macaroni and Cheese

(Ready in about 40 min | Servings 3 | Normal)

Ingredients:

- 1 and ½ cups of favorite macaroni

- Cooking spray

- ½ cup of heavy cream

- 1 cup of chicken stock

- ¾ cup of cheddar cheese, shredded

- ½ cup mozzarella cheese, shredded

- ¼ cup of parmesan, shredded

- Salt and black pepper to the taste

Directions:

1. Spray a pan with cooking spray, add macaroni, heavy cream, stock, cheddar cheese, mozzarella, and parmesan but also salt and pepper, toss well,

place pan in your AirFryer's basket, and cook for 30 minutes.

2. Divide among plates and serve for lunch.

Enjoy!

Nutrition: Calories: 341, Fat: 7g, Fiber: 8g, Carbs: 18g, Protein: 4g.

Conclusion

Air Fryers provide a much healthier method of frying food than conventional frying. However, it is necessary to take into account certain important aspects that cannot be ignored when using this small appliance.

Air Fryers are appliances that cook by circulating hot air around the food using the convection mechanism. In this type of fryer, also called air fryers, a mechanical fan circulates the hot air around the food.

The air fryer system causes a series of reactions that cause the food to darken. These reactions are twofold: caramelization and non-enzymatic *protein glycosylation (also called Maillard reaction).*

In caramelization, sugars are broken down and chemically transformed into complex brown substances. In the non-enzymatic protein glycosylation or Maillard reaction, the carbohydrates (sugars) and proteins in the food react with each other.

The result is the formation of certain compounds that give the food its flavor. Non-enzymatic glycosylation of proteins or Maillard reaction requires temperatures between 140 and 165 °C), while caramelization temperatures depend on the sugar to caramelize and vary from 110 to 180 °C.

Traditional frying methods induce non-enzymatic protein glycosylation or Maillard effect by completely submerging foods in hot oil, which reach much higher temperatures than boiling water.

Air Fryers, on the other hand, coat the food with a thin layer of oil while circulating heated air up to 200 °C, applying heat to initiate the reaction. In this way, the air fryer is able to produce fried food with its usual browned color, much less oil than a traditional fryer.

CPSIA information can be obtained
at www.ICGtesting.com
Printed in the USA
BVHW062038010321
601387BV00007B/499